Doctor's Little Book of Wisdom

Filled with Dr. Forgey's valuable tips gathered from his personal experiences being a family physician over 20 years.

By William W. Forgey, M.D.

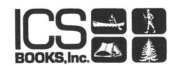

ICS BOOKS, Inc.
Merrillville, IN

Doctor's Little Book of Wisdom

Copyright © 1995 by William W. Forgey, M.D.

10 9 8 7 6 5 4 3 2 1

Published by:
ICS BOOKS, Inc
1370 E. 86th Place
Merrillville, IN 46410
800-541-7323

Printed in the U.S.A.
All ICS titles are printed on 50% recycled paper from
pre-consumer waste. All sheets are processed without
using acid.

Library of Congress Cataloging-in-Publication Data

Forgey, William W., 1942-
    Doctor's little book of wisdom / by William W. Forgey.
      p.   cm.
    ISBN 1-57034-016-1
    1.Medicine, Popular--Miscellanea   . I. Title.
RC82.F67 1995
610--dc20   95-8833
                                             CIP

Dedication

This book is fondly dedicated to those who taught me the craft and science of medicine and to my patients who constantly remind me of the humanity that makes it all worth while.

William W. Forgey, M.D.
Merrillville, Indiana

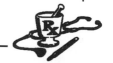

Foreword

There is an adage in medicine: "Never say never." This book has many "nevers" and some of the equally appropriate "always." These statements are generalized truths and should at least get you to pause and consider their potential importance in your life.

This is a book of prevention. As a physician I spend all too much of my time trying to patch up what amounts to a lack of prevention on the part of my patients. Knowing what to do to prevent a degradation of health frequently means knowing how to improve it, to maintain what we have, or to at least not accelerate unwittingly nature's tendency to batter us around.

But what form should this advice take?

I remember all too well the day I was counseling a young businessman on some of the hazards he would face on a trip to one of the developing nations. He came in for travel shots, yet infectious disease was probably the least important of the hazards that he was going to face, and most of the chance for catching an illness would have to be minimized by technique of living and not by a simple immunization. As I was providing him with a sheaf of printed materials and starting to explain them, he cut me short saying, "How long is this going to take?"

We infrequently wish to take the time to really learn about our health and safety. It is my hope that the format of this book will lend itself to easy, enjoyable reading. Perhaps it will be the best method of spreading information in a fun and interesting manner.

Possibly this book will be the best format for you to learn some valuable tips gathered from my personal experiences being a family physician over the past twenty years. Or, maybe it will provide you with the opportunity to provide a close friend or relative with this information in a fashion that they will enjoy and understand.

Best wishes and good health.

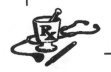

William W. Forgey, M.D.
Crown Point, Indiana

1. Loud music in earphones will damage hearing and result in chronic ear ringing.

2. Sun tanning ages your skin a year and a half for each summer of exposure.

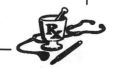

3. Install smoke alarms and check them every three months.

4. Visit someone in a nursing home at least monthly.

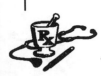

5. If you own firearms, store them unloaded in locked containers.

6. When anything irritating is splashed into your eye, irrigate immediately with large amounts of water.

7. Cool burns immediately with cold water.

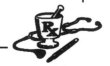

8.   A child is never too old to be kissed
      or hugged; you are never too old to
      kiss or hug your parent.

9.   If your spouse or significant other
      ever hits you once, dump 'em.

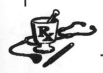

10. The incidence of lung cancer magically escalates after smoking a pack of cigarettes a day for 40 years.

11. Emphysema starts with the very first cigarette that you smoke.

12. Emphysema is never noticed on x-ray films until it is quite advanced.

13. Persons who smoke from their teenage years usually cannot walk to their mail box without a rest by the time they are 60 years old.

14. Antibiotics do not cure viral infections.

15. The more often that you take an antibiotic, the greater the chance that you will become allergic to it and not be able to use it in the future.

16. Do note confuse side effects of a medication with allergies to a medication. Allergies include the development of a rash, difficulty breathing, shock, or a fever due to the antibiotic. Most other adverse reactions are side effects and possibly will not prevent you from using that antibiotic again if necessary.

17. Volunteer to work in a hospital or nursing home – you will be surprised what you will learn about medicine, physicians, and humanity.

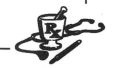

18. Never start the car motor before fastening your seat belt.

19. Never start the car motor until everyone else in the car has fastened their seat belt also.

20. Always use seat belts, especially in a taxicab.

21. Whenever you need to turn on your windshield wipers, turn on your headlights.

22. Always wear a helmet when you are riding a non-enclosed vehicle.

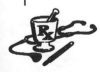

23.   Never treat viral fever in a child with aspirin.

24.   While not strictly necessary, it is never wrong to treat a fever with gentle cooling or medications such as acetaminophen (Tylenol®).

25.   Acetaminophen is a safe product properly used – but over-doses kill.

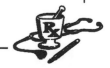

26. Always eat one meal a day as a family sitting down together. If this is not possible daily, do it at least once a week.

27. Do not allow the TV set to be running when having that meal.

28. Never have a pet that is stronger than one of your children.

29. Never have a coffee table, or similar low, sharp-edged furniture, when children younger than 7 years old are around to avoid split-open foreheads.

30. Never follow any medical advice, even
     from a book like this, without using
     common sense.

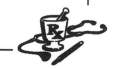

31.   A crawling child will aggressively try to enter cabinets and ground-level storage areas – place hazardous substances out of reach.

32.   A walking child can climb anywhere you can – lock hazardous substances.

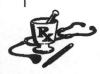

33. Learn how to perform CPR.

34. Always carry a one-way CPR mask in your purse or car for your safety when helping others.

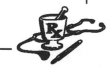

35.   Never chew on pens or small objects – use chewing gum instead.

36.   Never run or play any sports with your tongue hanging out of your mouth a la Michael Jordan – it might need to be reattached.

37.   Never lick a freezing-cold metal object.

38.   Taste only a small portion of liquid or food that is steaming hot to prevent mouth burns.

39.   Never smell the contents of a bottle by sniffing directly from the opening – wave the scent towards your nose with your free hand and sniff the air cautiously.

40.   Donate blood.

41.   Donate any usable tissue upon your death.

42.   Encourage others to do the same.

43.   Donate your remains to your state medical
       school for anatomical dissection by students.

44.   Obtain a living will.

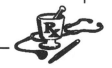

45.   Never try to cure a mouth sore by placing an aspirin tablet against it.

46.   Heat kills! Acclimatize by limiting initial exposure times and by drinking at least one eight-ounce glass of water every 20 minutes.

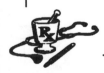

47. Attend free health fairs and blood pressure checks whenever you have the chance.

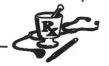

48. Never apply ice to a snake bite.

49. The best snake bite first aid is to use the Sawyer Extractor® first aid suction device immediately, then seek professional help.

50. Apply ice to bee stings.

51. The best bee sting first aid is to use the Sawyer Extractor first aid suction device immediately. If you have a history of severe allergic reactions to bee stings, also carry and know how to use an Anaguard®, Anakit®, or Epi-Pen® injectable kit and seek professional help. [1]

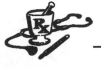

[1] The Sawyer Extractor® can be purchased at any camping or outdoor store.

52. Organize and check expiration dates in your medical kits and cabinets twice yearly.

53. Once medicine bottles have been opened, they may deteriorate faster than the expiration date indicates.

54. If food leaves a grease spot on paper, avoid eating it.

55. Virtually any bleeding can be stopped with direct pressure.

56. Never use over-the-counter nose drops more than three consecutive days to prevent rebound congestion and nose membrane irritation.

57. If you suffer from chronic foot or ankle pain, see a podiatrist.

58. The best preventative health investment is a consultation with a registered dietician.

59. When eating eggs, avoid the yolk.

60. All fruits and vegetables are good for you, except avocados.

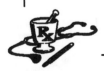

61. Asthma is usually caused by an allergy.

62. Antihistamines can prevent allergies, but too much drying action can worsen asthma.

63. Congestion without fever is caused by an allergy.

64. Antibiotics do not help treat allergies.

65. It is OK to treat congestion with over-the-counter medications only, unless accompanied by a fever that lasts longer than 24 hours.

66. Most headaches are caused by muscle spasm, generally from posture or neck problems.

67. Elevated blood pressure is almost never a cause of headache.

68. Elevated blood pressure usually has no symptoms – it is the silent killer.

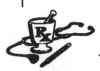

69. An average of five of your blood pressure readings should not be above 140 over 90.

70. The systolic, or upper BP reading, results when the heart contracts.

71. The diastolic, or lower BP reading, results between heart contractions.

72. Always check your blood pressure between doctor office visits. Some people have elevated blood pressures only in their doctor's office and might be over-medicated because of this.

73. Before visiting your doctor, make a written list of your concerns and show it to him - it is better than attempting to remember everything and it is faster for the doctor than reading items off one at a time.

74. The best question to ask about the necessity of a test is "Could the result change recommended therapy? If it would not, why take it?"

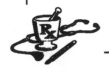

75. When looking for a new doctor, ask three pharmacists for three names. Choose a name that pops up more than once.

76. When looking for a new doctor, ask a hospital-employed nurse. A person in that position knows who is practicing good medicine with a decent personality.

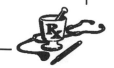

77.   Do not let abusive office staff deter you from using a good doctor – just complain to him.

78.   Do not ask to speak to the doctor if you are calling for an appointment.

79.   If you really want to speak to the doctor, but the staff won't let you, tell them you work for the hospital staff quality review committee.

80.   If it's really an emergency, don't bother calling the doctor, call 911.

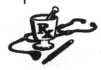

81.   Medical records are as much your property
        as they are the doctor's or the hospital's.

82.   Doctors may seem omnipotent, but they
        have all of the frailties of other humans – be
        patient, forgiving, or ask for a second
        opinion.

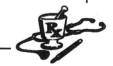

83. When in an auto accident, hope an EMT shows up and not a doctor.

84. When in an office and your symptoms are complex or seem serious, hope a doctor shows up and not a paramedical person.

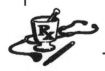

85.   Use cold on any new muscle or joint injury.

86.   The adage "If you can move it, it's not broken" is not true.

87.   Frequent vaginal douching should never be required.

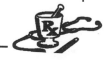

88. Use olive oil when cooking oil is required.

89. Poach fish, rather than frying.

90. When cooking meats, broil to decrease grease content.

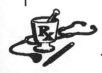

91. Clean wounds with copious irrigation.

92. Avoid alcohol, iodine, harsh soaps, or hydrogen peroxide when cleansing wounds.

93. After swimming or showering, dry your ear canals with sweet oil or after swim-drops such as Swim Ear®.

94. Never take any arthritis medicine on an empty stomach.

95. Never eat just before going to bed.

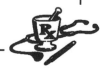

96.   Walk at least 1/2 hour three times a week.

97.   Avoid using any cleansing or polishing agent
        without adequate ventilation.

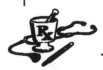

98.   Drink eight glasses of water daily.

99.   Drink one to three glasses of wine daily.

100.   Don't confuse the above recommendations.

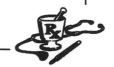

101. Take an aspirin every day.

102. Take vitamin A every day.

103. Never take megadoses of vitamins or use anything to excess.

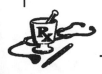

104. Exercise for 1/2 hour at least three times a week.

105. Encourage a friend to exercise with you.

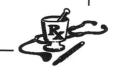

106. Keep a pair of fine pointed tweezers handy.

107. Wash your feet, using a washcloth, daily. Do not think a shower splashing on your feet actually cleans them.

108. Don't scratch an itch – apply cold instead.

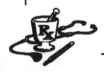

109. Try removing a foreign body from your eye by blinking under water.

110. Kill an insect stuck in your ear canal with several drops of cooking oil, then seek professional help to remove it.

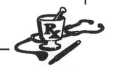

111.   If you don't know what to do,
        do what your mother would
        have done.

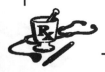

112. Use it or lose it – this applies to your brain, your muscle, and your libido.

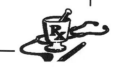

113. When on multiple medications, lay out the pills you need each day in the morning.

114. Always take over-the-counter aspirin or ibuprofen on a full stomach.

115. If a pill can be easily divided in half, have your doctor prescribe the medication at double the required strength. By taking 1/2 tablet you will cut your drug cost in half.

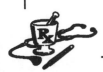

116. Always apply cold to new injuries and heat to injuries that occurred 24 hours or longer ago.

117. Never kiss a pet.

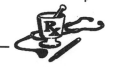

118.   Keep electrical equipment away from sinks and bath tubs.

119.   If you feel short of breath, take slow deep breaths and blow out against pursed lips, rather than taking rapid shallow breaths.

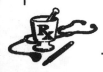

120. Never cross your legs as it decreases your leg circulation.

121. Sit on your bed for five minutes before getting up to walk after any rest period.

122. Install a telephone next to your bed.

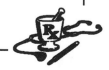

123.   Never salt your food without tasting it first.

124.   Never salt your food regardless.

125.   Avoid food preserved with nitrites.

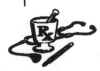

126.   Never walk barefoot in your house at night.

127.   Never walk barefoot outside.

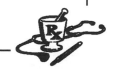

128. Never read in dim light.

129. Never read in direct sunlight.

130. Sleep with your windows open 1/2 inch.

131. Never try to pet a stray dog or cat.

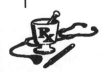

132.   If you catch on fire – stop, drop, and roll.

133.   Don't try to outrun a tornado – stop and drop.

134.   When lightning is nearby – stop and squat.

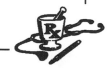

135.   Always use a stepladder, never a chair.

136.   When twenty years old you can safely fall a
distance equal to your height – subtract one
foot from this figure for every decade which
you age afterwards and never climb above
that distance.

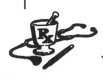

137.   Avoid constipation by drinking a warm and a cold beverage each morning; staying hydrated during the day; answering nature's call when you feel the urge – don't suppress it; and adding fruit and bulk to your diet.

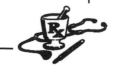

138. Don't go barefoot in public showers to avoid athlete's foot and plantar's warts.

139. To avoid callouses, wear gloves.

140. Always wear a lumbar support when lifting.

141. Always lift with your legs and not with your back.

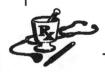

142.   Stretch out before working hard to avoid muscle injury.

143.   Stretch out after working hard to avoid muscle spasm.

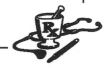

144. Always wear goggles or safety glasses when operating a machine, including a weed eater or lawn mower.

145. Always wear goggles or safety glasses when striking an object with another.

146. Never stick your hand into a garbage disposal unit or other machine that might gobble it up or squeeze it flat.

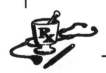

147.   Do not shut a door when anyone is nearby –
       someone may be trying to come through or
       in the act of sticking their hand in the
       opening.

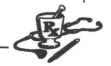

148. Do not wipe your eyes with your fingers.

149. Do not poke anything into your ear smaller than your elbow.

150. Do not pick your nose with anything – the nose harbors bacteria that are frequently harmless until you scratch them into your eye, ear, or skin.

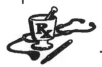

151. Don't press or prick acne as you may spread the germs. Use a benzoyl peroxide product instead.

152. If you have acne, avoid oily skin products, but also avoid drying the skin or abrading it. Use a mild soap such as Dove Unscented® or Neutrogena®.

153. To protect your skin from oily cosmetic buildup, use powder brushes and loose powders only on the face.

154. Food, such as chocolate or greasy foods, is seldom a cause of acne.

155. Avoid high doses of iodine in vitamins if you are prone to acne.

156.   Use an antihistamine to prevent allergies
        rather than trying to treat them.

157.   If you have allergies to outdoor pollens,
        wash your hair when coming inside.

158.   If you awaken at night with a severe
        sneezing or coughing allergy attack, take a
        hot shower to wash off allergens and to open
        your respiratory passages.

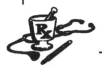

159. Wear sunglasses. They protect your eyes from ultraviolet rays and possible allergens and dust.

160. Do not allow anyone to smoke in your house, unless they sit on the fireplace hearth to draft the smoke up the chimney.

161. Do not burn chemically treated wood in your fireplace.

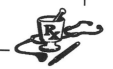

162. If you have allergies, keep your windows shut spring through fall, but crack them open during the winter.

163. To prevent allergies, dust with a damp cloth.

164. Use a dehumidifier to prevent mold from growing in your home or apartment.

165. If you are prone to allergies, leave the lawn mowing to someone else.

166. If you are allergic to animal dander, bathe your pet frequently.

167. If you have arthritis that results in stiffness and pain in the mornings, try sleeping in a sleeping bag on top of your bed – the warmth can relieve early morning ache.

168. If you gain ten pounds of weight, this results in 40 additional pounds of stress on your knees.

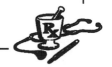

169. Keep the humidity in your home under 40% and over 20%.

170. Check houseplants for mold growth.

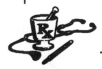

171. Remove your shoes when sitting at your desk or at any other time when possible.

172. Never wear the same pair of shoes two days in a row.

173. Severe itching from athlete's foot can be helped by soaking in a quart of warm water containing 6 black tea bags.

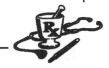

174. For acute back pain initially apply an
ice pack for 20 minutes, take it off for
30 minutes, then reapply for 20 minutes. After
24 hours apply heat for 20 minutes every
hour, have gentle massages, and take a
muscle relaxer and aspirin or ibuprofen.

175. If sitting for a long time is bothering your
low back, make a chair back support by
rolling a towel into the circumference of
your forearm.

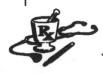

176. Bad breath problem? Try cleaning your tongue, flossing then rinsing your mouth, and munching on parsley.

177. To prevent excessive belching, avoid carbonated beverages, avoid belches as they automatically cause air swallowing, eat slowly, and treat nasal congestion.

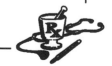

178.   Treat itching from bites, chicken pox, or plant allergies with calamine lotion – it's effective, cheap, and safe.

179.   Use ice packs on small areas that itch severely 20 minutes at a time as needed.

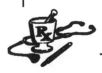

180. Remove ticks with sharp pointed tweezers, grasping as close to the skin as possible, even nipping a piece of local skin if necessary. Local skin is normally anesthetized and the removal is painless.

181. Ticks have to be on your body about 6 hours before they attach.

182. Ticks have to be attached over 24 hours to give Lyme disease to their host.

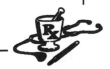

183. Do not avoid urinating if possible. Always go when the urge hits.

184. Urinate within 15 minutes of having sexual intercourse.

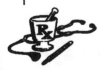

185. In case of abdominal pain, it is always proper to apply a heating pad.

186. If you have a fever, rest in bed.

187. Prolonged sitting can lead to hemorrhoids and varicose veins.

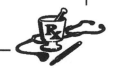

188. Cover friction blisters and hot spots with a gel-type dressing such as Spenco 2nd Skin®, sold in most pharmacies.

189. When opening painful blisters, use a sharp blade sterilized in alcohol and cut sufficiently to promote adequate collapse of the blister dome.

190. Leave the top of a blister on, unless it becomes white and puffy; then simply cut it off.

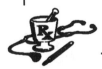

191. Women with tender breasts should avoid caffeine, nicotine, and chocolate – all of which aggravate fibrocystic breast development.

192. Vitamin E taken at 800 IU per day may help prevent tenderness in fibrocystic breasts.

193. Ibuprofen is the best over-the-counter drug treatment for fibrocystic breasts.

194. If breasts become tender during or just before menses, avoid salt to help reduce fluid retention.

195. To minimize bruising after injury,
      immediately apply cold – such as ice
      wrapped in a damp cloth – 10 to 20 minutes,
      repeating every hour, but changing to heat
      after 24 hours.

196. Rest bruised areas, with elevation
      when possible.

197. Place a rubber mat in your bathtub or
      shower and have a sturdy handhold.

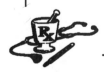

198.   Do not put butter on burns.

199.   Never open a radiator cap on a hot motor.

200.   Do not spray lighter fluid on charcoal that has already been lit.

201.   Do not use white gas (naphtha, or Coleman fuel) to start a fire.

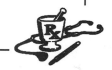

202. Open packaged microwave foods carefully and pointed away from your face to prevent steam burns.

203. Never pour hot fluids into containers on your lap or when someone is holding them.

204. Keep handles on pots cooking on the stove turned inward, away from the stove edge.

205. Keep your hot water heater set lower then 120° F (49° C).

206.   Do not smoke in bed.

207.   Install carbon monoxide detectors that
       digitally detect and report all levels of CO to
       better control intake of this incidious killer.

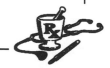

208.   Don't overload electric outlets.

209.   Cover unused electrical outlets with caps, especially with children around.

210.   Keep matches and lighters away from a child's reach – and that includes your purse, not just the kitchen cabinet.

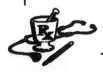

211.   Off limits to kids:

Garbage cans
Toilet bowls
Stoves
Cleanser storage areas
Toolboxes
Electrical switches
Medicine cabinet
Guns and ammunition
Knife storage area
Mark these areas with "Mr. Uck" signs!

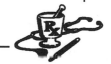

212. Teach kids how to dial 911 or 0 and give their name and location (or to read the telephone number from the phone they are using).

213. Learn or post the telephone number of the local poison control center (normally your local hospital emergency room – check with them).

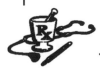

214.　　Have home fire drills.

215.　　Have a private hotel fire drill for your family
　　　　when traveling.

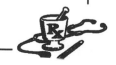

216. At check-in, ask if your hotel room is equipped with smoke and carbon monoxide detectors.

217. Do not stay above the 7th floor for easier fire rescue or below the 3rd floor for greater security from outside room invasion.

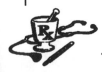

218.   Treat canker sores with Orabase with
        Benzocaine® or ask your doctor for a Rx of
        Kenalog in Orabase®.

219.   If a mouth sore doesn't heal within three
        weeks, see your dentist or doctor.

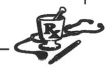

220.   Several things can cause tingling and
       numbness and/or pain of the hand and wrist,
       but a very common cause is carpal tunnel
       syndrome.

221.   Carpal tunnel syndrome can be treated by
       proper wrist splinting, ergomatic
       positioning, ice to the wrist and forearm 5 to
       15 minutes three times a day, appropriate
       rest, ibuprofen, exercise, or surgery – your
       choice but do something when the
       symptoms start or you'll end up with the last
       choice.

222. Chafing can be prevented with powders, creams, or ointments – I prefer Vaseline®.

223. Avoid licking chapped lips – use frequent applications of lip balm or good old Vaseline®.

224. Use sunscreen on your lips as well as your skin.

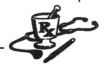

225. Drink at least 8 ounces of fluid every two hours when ill – the best fluid: chicken soup!

226. Rest when ill.

227. Fever over 102°F (39° C), severe headache or sore throat, or symptoms that persist over 36 hours are reasons to seek professional help.

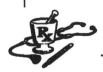

228. Gargle every one to two hours with salt water to treat a sore throat, but don't make it too strong. Use one level teaspoon to one quart of water.

229. Stuffy nose? Flush with dilute salt water – 3 or 4 sprays, 5 to 6 times daily.

230. Smoking aggravates cold symptoms – it's a great time to try to stop!

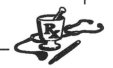

231. A major reason people do not try to stop smoking is the fear of failure. So what if you fail a dozen times? Try, try again.

232. Once you have stopped smoking, you are still a smoker – keep your guard up. It's all too easy to fall off the wagon and start again. Be especially careful during times of stress and various anniversaries of the day you stopped.

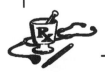

233. Do not talk on the telephone during an electrical storm.

234. Do not stand near fences, trees, or anything higher than you during an electrical storm.

235. If you are golfing during an electrical storm, don't.

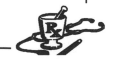

236. Unplug your computer and television during an electrical storm.

237. Avoid bathing or having contact with plumbing and water pipes during an electrical storm.

238. If you see someone struck by lightning and they appear dead, call 911 and perform CPR until relieved.

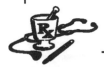

239.   When an acquaintance makes either strongly positive or negative comments about a physician, before accepting their view, consider what you know about the informant's ability to judge. Would you accept their advice on choosing your lawyer, husband, wife?

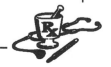

240. Do not over-diagnosis constipation. A bowel movement every two to three days is normal for some people.

241. Treat constipation with exercise, eight cups of fluid daily, 20 to 35 grams of fiber daily, and going when you feel the urge.

242. Eat seven servings of fruits and vegetables and six to eleven servings of grain products daily.

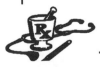

243. If you have dandruff, choose a shampoo that contains zinc pyrithione, selenium sulfide, sulfur, or salicylic acid and rotate them monthly.

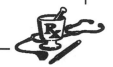

244.   If you *must* scratch an itch, use the pads of your fingers, not your hands.

245.   For skin allergy, take an over-the-counter antihistamine, but be cautious when applying antihistamine ointments – they tend to be a *cause* of skin allergy.

246.   Also, "-caine" ointments tend to be sensitizing and can increase itch and irritation.

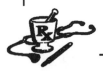

247. An oatmeal bath can help the itch of chicken pox – make it by filling a handkerchief with a cup of oatmeal, tie it into a ball, and swish in tepid water.

248. Avoid contact with hot water when you have a skin irritation.

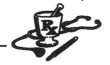

249. When working in weeds or brush, wear a long-sleeve shirt and work gloves, even if you are not yet sensitive to plants.

250. We are not born allergic to plants, but with exposure 50 percent of the population will acquire an allergy.

251. Many people are allergic to pine and fir needles if they are poked by them – be careful taking the Christmas tree down.

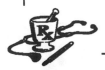

252. Know how to recognize the common forms of poison ivy, oak, and sumac.

253. Plant allergies can spread by smoke and contact with contaminated clothing, tools, and pet fur.

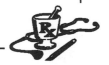

254. Wash all new clothes before wearing. Some chemicals used in manufacturing can cause skin allergy.

255. Keep your fingernails and toenails trimmed.

256. Whether in a lake or pool, wash after swimming.

257. When your head becomes wet, dry your ears thoroughly and consider using a drying variety of ear drop or make a mixture of hydrogen peroxide and sweet oil and use four drops per side.

258.   A modern disaster --> protect your family
       from increased ultraviolet light exposure.[2]

259.   Avoid the sun between 10:00 a.m. and
       3:00 p.m., when the sun's rays are the most
       damaging to your skin.

[2] Obtain a copy of *Ozone, UV, and Your Health* by Buck Tilton and Roger Cox, ICS Books,
$6.99

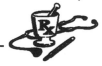

260. Over 12 million Americans develop diabetes during their life. Watch for the signs such as frequent urination accompanied by unusual thirst, extreme hunger, and at times rapid weight loss, easy tiring, weakness, and fatigue.

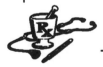

261.   Never place an object in your mouth to chew
       on and lie down – you may fall asleep and
       risk a chance of aspiration.

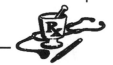

262. Diaper rash should always clear with treatment in a few days.

263. To avoid diaper rash, keep the baby dry and use super-absorbent diapers.

264. To treat diaper rash, take the diaper off.

265. Very angry diaper rash may be due to a yeast infection and should readily clear with the use of an anti-fungal cream such as miconazole 2%. Hint – purchase the vaginal cream, three times the product for only twice the cost.

266. Diarrhea caused by a virus can start within hours, from bacteria within days, from parasites (such as giardia) from one to four weeks.

267. Diarrhea from a virus can last days; from bacteria, weeks; and from parasites, months.

268. Besides infection, diarrhea can be caused by lactose (milk) intolerance, wheat intolerance, irritable bowel syndrome, Crohn's disease or ulcerative colitis, illnesses ranging from diabetes to thyroid disorders, and cancer.

269.   Over-bathing can dry skin.

270.   Hot water tends to dry your skin more than cool water.

271.   Moisturize dry skin with a lotion or cream right after bathing while your skin is still damp.

272.   If using a bath oil to moisturize your skin, be careful that you or the next person using the tub doesn't slip.

273.   Ear pain can sometimes be due to problems with your temporomandibular joint (TMJ), teeth, throat, tonsils, or tongue.

274.   Hearing loss associated with an ear infection is usually temporary, but untreated can result in permanency.

275. If you are congested and have ear pain, the source may be in the inner ear and ear drops will be of no help – you will require a decongestant and possibly an antibiotic.

276. If you have ear pain and it hurts to pull on the ear lobe or push on the tragus (the flap in front of your ear), you probably have a swimmer's ear that can be relieved by ear drops.

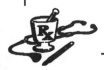

277.   When a young child is running a fever or
       vomiting, it is possible that he or she has a
       severe ear infection.

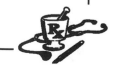

278. Protect your eyes with goggles when swimming.

279. Protect your eyes from direct and reflected light. Reflected ultraviolet light causes damage.

280. When reading, avoid extremes of too much or too little light.

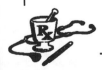

281. A fever probably helps the body fight infection, but cool the patient when it goes over 103°F (39°C).

282. Do not bundle up when you have a fever.

283. If you have a fever and are chilling, try to use the least amount of covers possible (compatible with comfort).

284. Do not give aspirin to a child with fever – use acetaminophen instead; it's safer.

285. Treat a hangnail by cutting it off with a sharp scissors and applying an antibiotic ointment.

286. Try to suppress a dry cough – it only causes additional bronchial irritation and continued coughing.

287. When ill use a vaporizer rather than a humidifier to increase the moisture in the air.

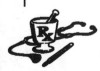

288. If you suffer from heartburn, avoid tomatoes and anything made from them.

289. Persons with a history of ulcers or having heartburn should avoid tomatoes, coffee, alcohol, or any spicy foods.

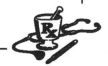

290. When choosing meat, always buy "select" which is 15 to 20% fat, as opposed to "choice" at 30 to 40% fat or "prime" at 40 to 45% fat by weight.

291. Avoid egg yolks, poultry skin, and pastry to cut your fat consumption.

292. Purchase and use a home blood pressure monitor.

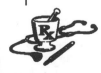

293.   Eat less salt.

294.   Exercise.

295.   Lose weight.

296.   Relax.

297.   Buy shoes that fit.

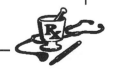

298.   Do not scratch an itch – cool it.

299.   Avoid applying heat to an itch or rash.

300.   Calamine lotion can help itches, but it does not treat hives.

301.   Dry, itchy skin needs to be moisturized.

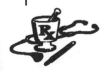

302.   If you develop hives and your voice
       becomes hoarse, seek emergency medical
       help as your airway may be closing off.

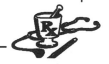

303. Lift out ingrown hairs using a straight pin or needle – do not gouge the skin.

304. Shave in the same direction each day to prevent hairs from curling and becoming ingrown.

305. Do not shave too closely – it is hard on your skin.

306. If you have insomnia, avoid naps during the
      day, take a hot bath before bedtime, read
      until tired, and try not to worry about it.

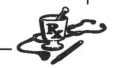

307. Menstrual cramps are better treated with ibuprofen or aspirin than with acetaminophen.

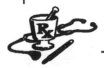

308.   If you easily get motion sickness in a car, it's best to be the driver and not the rider.

309.   Don't try to read in a car if you tend to have motion sickness.

310.   If muscle cramps are a frequent problem, try a water workout or swimming for exercise.

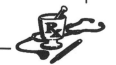

311. Learn your limits.

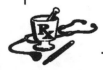

312. If you feel like you might vomit, don't try to initially prevent it. Persistent vomiting can be treated with prescription medications, a cold compress to your head, taking clear liquids, and trying Pepto-Bismol®.

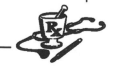

313. If your teeth are sensitive, brush with a desensitizing toothpaste after each meal, use a fluoride mouth rinse and see your dentist.

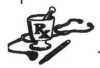

314. When shaving, moisten your skin before applying shaving foam for better results.

315. If you have razor burn, stop shaving as close and use an over-the-counter hydrocortisone cream to soothe your face.

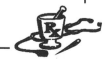

316. Pinching your nostrils closed will stop most nosebleeds and works better than any other technique.

317. If you have chronic nosebleeds, avoid aspirin.

318. Treat chronic nosebleeds with hydration, humidify your room, and use saline spray in your nose frequently.

319. Calm a child with a nosebleed as crying increases the blood flow and sniffling decreases basal blood clotting.

320. If you have chronic nosebleeds, increase your iron intake.

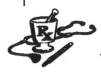

321. If you have oily skin, use only water-based cosmetics; if you have dry skin, use oil-based products.

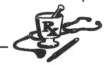

322.   Prevent osteoporosis with walking, adequate
        calcium intake, replacing hormones after
        menopause, and decreasing salt, nicotine,
        alcohol, and caffeine intake.

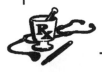

323. Avoid decongestant nasal sprays.

324. Use a fluoride rinse daily.

325. Floss.

326. A painful tooth can be treated by applying oil of cloves, or covering with a piece of sugarless chewing gum until you can reach a dentist.

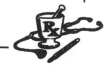

327. Treat shin splints by wrapping the lower leg in a compression bandage while exercising.

328. Treat a "stitch in the side" by poking deeply into the sore area with your finger tips, then purse your lips tightly and blow out forcefully.

329. Decrease snoring by sleeping on your side or with your head elevated.

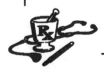

330. Stop snoring by waking the offending person up – well almost. Just a gentle nudge will frequently do the trick, for a while.

331. Read labels – compute the amounts of fat and cholesterol which you are eating.

332. Your total fat intake should be less than 30% of the calories which you are eating.

333. Saturated fat should be less than 10% of your daily calorie intake.

334. Cholesterol intake should be less than 300 mg per day.

Physical Examination Guidelines

1. Know the risk factors for developing blood vessel blockage: obesity, family history of disease, use of tobacco, family history of heart or other blood vessel blockage, untreated high blood pressure, high cholesterol, and/or high triglyceride.

2. Have your doctor listen to your carotid arteries (neck) after the age of 40 if you have symptoms of a stroke or increased risk of blood vessel blockage.

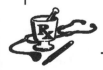

Physical Examination Guidelines

3.   Have a dental examination annually after the age of 18, if you drink alcohol or use tobacco products, to check for mouth cancer.

4.   Your body skin surface should be inspected visually by a physician after the age of 18 if you have had a history of sunburns.

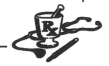

Physical Examination Guidelines

5.   Women 18 years and older should have a yearly breast examination if breast cancer occurred before menopause in a first-degree relative.

6.   All women should have a breast examination by their physician yearly after the age of 40.

7.   A PAP smear should be taken yearly starting at the age of first intercourse in women with high risk: early age of first intercourse or multiple sexual partners.

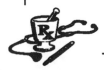

Physical Examination Guidelines

8.   In women at average risk, a PAP smear every third year confers 96 percent of the benefit of annual screening.

9.   A routine thyroid test should be ordered on all women at age 60

10.   Men should have their prostates checked at age 40 every two years and then yearly after the age of 50 to evaluate enlargement and for cancer screening.

Physical Examination Guidelines

11. Your blood pressure should be taken at each physician visit.

12. Have your child's eyesight examined at school entry and at least every three years while in school.

13. Young adults should have eyesight examined every 5 years.

14. At age 65, have eyesight examined yearly.

Physical Examination Guidelines

15.   A full audiometry hearing test should be obtained at age 18 and 65 routinely and annually between the ages of 19 and 64 if you are exposed to loud noises, including indiscriminate choice in music over earphones.

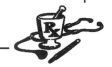

Physical Examination Guidelines

16. Have your stool tested yearly for evidence of microscopic blood (Hemoccult) as a colon cancer screen.

17. Flexible sigmoidoscopy every ten years can significantly reduce your chance of dying from colon cancer.

18. Take an aspirin daily after the age of 40 if you have a high risk of artery disease or family history of heart disease and no risk of stroke or bleeding.

Physical Examination Guidelines

19. Ladies should take estrogen and progesterone if they have a high risk of heart blood vessel blockage or a high risk of osteoporosis; avoid taking this if there is an above-average risk of breast cancer.

20. Ladies with a uterus taking estrogen should also take progesterone to reduce the chance of inducing cervical cancer.

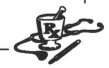

Physical Examination Guidelines

21. The US Preventative Services Task Force recommends a urine analysis on persons at age 60 and routinely on diabetic patients.

22. Persons with a family history of diabetes and marked obesity should have routine fasting blood sugar tests.

23. Routine fasting cholesterol screening should be performed every five years after the age of 30.

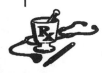

Physical Examination Guidelines

24. Routine HIV (AIDS) testing should be done on anyone over the age of 18 who has a high risk behavior (sexual promiscuity or IV drug use) and once on people who had received transfusions between 1978-1985.

25. Routine syphilis tests are not needed unless a person engages in high risk-sexual activity.

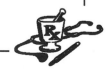

Physical Examination Guidelines

26. Resting electrocardiograms are not routinely of value, unless the person is over 40 years of age with risk factors for cardiac artery blockage or if they are about to start an exercise program.

27. A glaucoma check should be made on everyone over the age of 65.

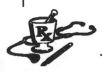

Physical Examination Guidelines

28. A TB test should be taken by persons if exposed, if taking high doses of steroids, or if they are HIV positive.

29. The American College of Physicians states that routine chest x-rays are not useful in saving lives, even in smokers. By the time a cancer is seen, it is too late. And emphysema is a given.

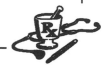

30.   A bone mineral analysis (an x-ray study) should be done in women approaching menopause, slender women, and women considering taking estrogen to prevent osteoporosis.

31.   A mammography should be done yearly in all women age 50 and older.

32.   Mammographies should be done above age 35 if there is a history of premenopausal breast cancer in a first degree relative.

Physical Examination Guidelines

33. Hepatitis B vaccine is very safe and should be obtained by everyone. This is a three-shot series and usually provides immunity for at least three years.

34. The Pneumococcal 23-valent vaccine should be obtained by everyone 65 years old or above. This is given as a single shot and usually provides immunity for at least 10 years.

35. Influenza vaccine should be obtained yearly by everyone 65 years or older.

36. Diphtheria-tetanus vaccine should be obtained by everyone each ten years.

Warnings that you should seek medical attention

Infection or skin irritation that persists

Bruising without injury

Sores that don't improve within a week or heal within two weeks

A rash that worries you

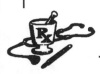

Warnings that you should seek medical attention

Increased urinary frequency:
with fever
with backache
with blood in urine
with weight loss
with recent injury
with discharge
male, over age 50
persists over 2 days

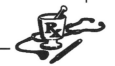

Warnings that you should seek medical attention

Breast with:
a lump or firmness
soreness on one side
a change in self-exam
nipple discharge on one side

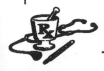

Warnings that you should seek medical attention

Persistent bad breath

Difficulty breathing or wheezing

Cough up blood

Dry cough for more than 10 days

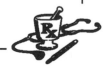

Warnings that you should seek medical attention

Adult with a fever above 103, or child above 102, for more than 24 hours

Fever with headache and stiff neck

Fever with sore throat

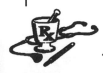

Warnings that you should seek medical attention

Cuts:
on the face
very deep or too dirty to clean
jagged
wider than 1/4 inch
infected (redness, red streaks, swelling, pus,
enlarged lymph nodes)
can't stop bleeding with direct pressure

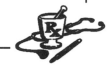

Warnings that you should seek medical attention

Signs of diabetes:
frequent urination with thirst
extreme hunger
rapid weight loss with weakness
persistent nausea, vomiting
blurred vision or change in sight
frequent skin infection
slow healing
vaginitis
impotence

Warnings that you should seek medical attention

Blood in stool

Diarrhea lasting longer than 2 days

Ear ache, drainage, or decreased hearing

Eye redness, pain, or vision change

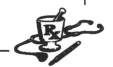

Warnings that you should seek medical attention

Paralysis

Weakness in a limb

Trouble swallowing

Persistent hiccups

Change in bowel patterns

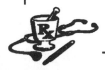

Warnings that you should seek medical attention

Laryngitis persisting more than 72 hours

Change in frequency or intensity of menstrual cramps

Pregnancy

Leg cramps when walking or at night

Frequent nosebleeds

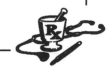

Warnings that you should seek medical attention

Resistant acne

Change in a "mole" color or size

Mucus that turns green or yellow or is associate with facial pain

Dental decay, change in gum color or swelling, tooth pain lasting longer than one hour

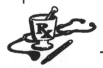

Warnings that you should seek medical attention

Sunburn that has extensive blistering, accompanied with fever and chills, pain or itching increases after 24 hours

Bleeding gums

Genital lesions, pain, or discharge

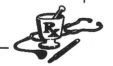

Warnings that you should seek medical attention

Vaginal discharge that is:
thin or foamy
grey to yellow-green
associated with abdominal pain
bloody between periods
bloody after menopause
recurrent
persisting over two weeks with treatment

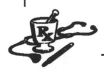

Warnings That Your Baby Requires Medical Attention

Diaper rash that lasts 2 days without improving or longer than 5 days

Rash that persists or spreads to arms, legs, or trunk

Fever over 101 or lasting more than 24 hours

Red eye or pus in eye

Pulling on an ear

Refuses to nurse or take a bottle

Vomiting or diarrhea

Failure to gain weight on a weekly basis

Not moving limbs equally well

Blood coming from a body opening

Unusually fussy or lethargic

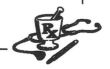

Look for these other Little Books of Wisdom at your
favorite bookstore or outdoor retailer

Camping's Little Book of Wisdom
By Dave Scott
ISBN 0-934802-96-3 $5.95
&
Teacher's Little Book of Wisdom
By Bob Algozzine
ISBN 1-57034-017-X $5.95

Look for Bachelor's and Traveler's Little Books of Wisdom
in the future